TREESOFHOPE

Facts of Life For Parents of Teens: Sex Education Curriculum For Parents of Teens Ages 13+
This First Edition Published in 2023 by
    Trees of Hope, 3901 West Broward Blvd., #122195,
    Fort Lauderdale, FL 33312
    www.treesofhope.org

ISBN 979-8-9885030-4-0

Copyright © Trees of Hope, 2023

All rights reserved. No part of this publication may be reproduced, stored in or introduced into a retrieval system, or transmitted, in any form, or by any means (electrical, mechanical, photocopying, recording or otherwise) without the prior written permission of the publisher. Any person who does any unauthorized act in relation to this publication may be liable to criminal prosecution and civil claims for damages.

Unless otherwise noted Scripture quotations are from THE HOLY BIBLE, NEW INTERNATIONAL VERSION®, NIV® Copyright © 1973, 1978, 1984, 2011 by Biblica, Inc.™ Used by permission. All rights reserved worldwide.

Author: Trees of Hope
Designed by Nicole Escobar

Visit treesofhope.org for any further information.

LIBRARY OF CONGRESS PUBLISHER'S CATALOGING-IN-PUBLICATION DATA
Names: Escobar, Nicole, designer. | Trees of Hope (Organization), issuing body.

Title: *Facts of Life For Parents of Teens: Sex Education Curriculum For Parents of Teens Ages 13+* / written by Trees of Hope; designed by Nicole Escobar.

Description: Fort Lauderdale, FL : published by Trees of Hope, [2023] | Series: Facts of life (Trees of Hope) ; v. 3.

Identifiers: ISBN: 979-8-9885030-4-0

Subjects: LCSH: Sex instruction--Study and teaching--Parent participation. | Sex instruction for teenagers--Study and teaching. | Sex instruction for teenagers--Religious aspects--Christianity--Study and teaching. | Teenagers--Sexual behavior--Religious aspects--Christianity--Study and teaching. | Puberty--Study and teaching. | Parenting. | Parenting--Religious aspects--Christianity.

Classification: LCC: HQ57 .F333 2023 | DDC: 649/.65--dc23

Facts of Life For Parents of Teens

SEX EDUCATION CURRICULUM FOR PARENTS OF TEENS AGES 13+

WRITTEN BY TREES OF HOPE
DESIGNED BY NICOLE ESCOBAR

PUBLISHED BY

TREESOFHOPE

LEARN MORE ABOUT THE MINISTRY TREES OF HOPE

Research shows that approximately 25% of the U.S. population has experienced sexual abuse at some point in their lives. Victims of childhood sexual abuse are far more likely to struggle with addiction, eating disorders, suicidal thoughts, and other destructive behaviors, and may even end up becoming abusers themselves. While the statistics are shocking and the effects disturbing, there is hope! Experts agree that 95% of childhood sexual abuse is preventable through education and training. That is where Trees of Hope comes in.

Trees of Hope was founded in 2006 by a sexual abuse survivor. Since that time, we have impacted thousands of people's lives through our prevention workshops and healing studies.

While we are humbled by what we've accomplished so far, there is still so much to be done. Children need to be protected from becoming victims in the future, and survivors need to heal from the wounds of their past. Trees of Hope will not stop until the scourge of sexual abuse has been completely and permanently eradicated from our world.

The ministry of Trees of Hope fights the silent epidemic of sexual abuse by following a two-fold organizational model composed of prevention and healing.

Regarding prevention, we offer free prevention workshops for parents, teachers, volunteers, and ministry leaders, along with educational resources designed to educate adults on identifying and preventing childhood sexual abuse. Workshops are carried out in-person, virtually, or prerecorded online, to suit the individual and their needs.

In our healing program, we aim to walk alongside those affected by sexual abuse by offering healing support groups three times a year by means of our church partnerships, individual studies, and online studies that can be taken at any time. We feel there should be no justification for any victim being unable to find healing. Accordingly, our unique curriculum is designed for a diverse range of specific needs, genders, and ages.

WELCOME TO THE FACTS OF LIFE SERIES

Bringing new life into the world is one of the most beautiful miracles the earth will ever witness. Is there anything more meaningful than children who look to you with complete trust for their needs, knowing they are safe within your care?

Children with loving, attentive parents begin their years of development in a safe environment that reflects family values and feelings of security and love.

Unfortunately, not every home has healthy relationships or values, leading to situations where many children have to attempt to navigate life without solid direction. One glance at society reveals the desperate need for spiritual revival within the family home.

As children age, outside influences and experiences will introduce countless new ideas to expand their knowledge and encourage them to explore the world around them. Some of these influences will come from events and people who share your family values. Additionally, others will, of course, occur through encounters with acquaintances who have sadly only known the hardships of figuring life out independently.

When the inevitable blending of both types of influence reaches your children, human reasoning may lead them to confusion and questions about the values taught in your home. Romantically loving a person of the same sex and choosing which sex they want to be may seem harmless to young people who are surrounded by the forceful push to accept these things.

What is less known about such topics is the increased suicide rate, necessary long-term counseling, the bypassing of emotional trauma that impacts those lifestyle choices, preexisting mental disorders, and many other negative factors.

The loving God who created every person is the God of order and peace. His perfect design creates each human being without error. Genesis 5:1-2 tells us: "...When God created human beings, he made them to be like himself. He created them male and female, and he blessed them and called them human." From the time each person is created and with every intricate detail carved out by the Master Creator, God has a plan for every human being.

As parents, you are your children's greatest influence.

In this invaluable series, each unit builds upon the previous unit, giving you solid concepts to help you teach your child important lessons about their bodies. This series is meant to be a help and a blessing to you. It is certainly not intended to highlight any inadequacies you may feel about your own personal knowledge. Teaching your children about sexual things may feel awkward, but the importance of children learning about these topics with godly values and correct teaching must supersede that discomfort.

Without further ado, you got this! We will walk with you every step of the way.

Let's jump in!

REFRESHER AND INTRODUCTION

If you've read the first two books in this three-book series, this book builds on the concepts and information shared in them. If you haven't read the second book, which covers topics that pertain to children between the ages of 6 and 10, below is an overview which shares the highlights.

WHAT CHILDREN SHOULD KNOW ABOUT MALE AND FEMALE BODIES, AND GOD'S DESIGN FOR MARRIAGE

Between the ages of 6-10, children should know the proper names for their genitals and that it is not okay for anyone to touch their private parts.

Maintaining an ongoing conversation about topics related to sexuality that lasts year after year helps the conversation to be more comfortable, natural, and open to the questions your children will have. Allowing them to ask questions and having a calm demeanor is important. You are their greatest teacher and will give them godly direction as their understanding about their bodies and sexuality develops. There is no shame in saying you don't know the answers to some of their questions but will find them.

You can teach this age group the differences between men's and women's reproductive organs. Learning the basics may initiate greater curiosity about their body parts. Basic answers to children's questions are usually enough at this age. You can give more information as they mature.

The modern society in which we live has a diverse variety of ideas about love, sex, and marriage that are different from God's design. Some of the ideas arise from an agenda pushed by elements of society that results in lifelong devastation for many people.

There is no criticism of the victims of broken families or those who have been fooled into believing things that are prevalent in the culture or society in which they find themselves. That being said, God's design for families is to unite a man and woman who love each other and have kept their bodies pure until marriage. When they've vowed to commit to each other and are wed, a healthy, loving relationship will bring forth children. It is then God's desire that those children be raised in a loving home that honors Him.

Because many alternative lifestyles (Some that even include young children) are widely expressed in our communities, classrooms will include children who are transgender. Some families will also have same-sex parents. Simple explanations will be necessary. Reminding children to always practice kindness, because some people do not know God's design for families, should also be mentioned. Children should be reassured that God made them perfect in the body they were born with.

EARLY PUBERTY

Most children go through puberty around 11 or 12, but some can begin as early as six years old for girls, or nine years old for boys. If your child begins developing pubic hair or growth in their private parts very early, you should speak to your doctor about what is happening.

When you notice puberty starting in your children, regular positive affirmations should be consistently given. This will offset any teasing from peers and help them understand that their bodies are growing as they should.

Normal and abnormal sexual behaviors

There are normal sexual behaviors your children will often display, which is a part of growing up and becoming aware of their own bodies. There are also abnormal behaviors that children may display, which indicates other things they may be seeing or experiencing. Your proper response to each type of sexual behavior is crucial. Overreacting can cause undue shame that can hinder healthy sexual development. When children display abnormal sexual behaviors, they are often unaware that they are doing anything abnormal.

Normal behaviors include:

- Having many sexually related questions, including those about pregnancy and menstruating

REFRESHER AND INTRODUCTION

- Curiosity about their peers' bodies (within their own age group and of the same sex), touching peers
- Experiencing sexual arousal and masturbating
- Talking about sexuality with peers
- Accidentally accessing pornography

Abnormal behaviors can be the result of being exposed to pornography (either accidentally or on purpose), seeing adults in sexual activity, family violence, loss of a loved one, and/or emotional neglect.

Some abnormal sexual behaviors include:

- Knowing about specific sexual activities and more information about sexuality than what is considered normal for their age
- Sexual behaviors that involve children with an age gap of four or more years
- Pressuring or forcing others into sexual behaviors
- Masturbating until they injure their genitals
- Publicly touching themselves or exposing themselves in public
- Rubbing their genitals on other people

If abnormal behaviors continue after you have calmly spoken to your children about them, you should keep track of the behavior and speak to your physician about your concerns.

TEACHING CHILDREN BODILY RESPECT FOR THEMSELVES AND OTHERS

Self-care helps children both physically and mentally, privately, and socially. As a parent, your own examples of good hygiene and healthy habits are important models. Children are more likely to follow your lead and not your words alone.

Continue welcoming any questions they may have and keep the conversation open during their growing years. You can mention changes you notice to help facilitate helpful conversations.

Help your children understand that there are negative consequences to poor personal hygiene. This would include issues such as bodily odor, tooth decay, bad breath, and being more susceptible to viruses and infections. Checking on your children's routines and making them more appealing (such as playing a two minute teeth-brushing song from the internet, and/or buying kids flavored toothpaste) can help as they develop healthy hygiene habits.

Children who are taught that their bodies are special and deserve proper care are more likely to develop healthy boundaries for their own bodies and for others'. When children respect themselves, they are less likely to allow others to treat them poorly. This is very helpful when your children are searching for a companion when they are older.

Teaching your children to treat others the way they want to be treated will help them understand that others have personal boundaries too. They can learn to respect others who may not be comfortable with certain physical touches, or who may want to keep some of their emotions private.

PARENTAL BOUNDARIES

Children should have healthy boundaries in their homes that teach and offer respect, and an environment that is greatly focused upon for the overall well-being of the entire family.

Children resent having no boundaries or rules, even when they sometimes push against them. However, those boundaries should be limited to what is necessary. The rules should be for the purpose of helping children learn responsibility, self-control, respect, and how to live more peacefully with others.

Making the rules clear, writing them down and posting them in the home, allowing the children to give some input, and keeping the list to what is necessary will encourage participation, which is the ultimate purpose and goal.

REFRESHER AND INTRODUCTION

TEACHING YOUR CHILDREN SEX-ED

Children will pick up many ideas about sexuality through peers, television, music, the internet, and other surrounding influences. Most will not offer God's view on the topic, which makes your input and teaching essential.

Remembering to stay calm when questions arise (even shocking questions) gives you the best chance of your children coming to you for answers, rather than fearing your response and finding their information from other people and places.

Age-appropriate books can help you with some of the questions your children will ask. Simple answers to many questions will be enough to satisfy their curiosity. You can give additional information when they ask.

Expect questions like: "Where do babies come from?" A sufficient response would be: "A man has millions of seeds, called sperm, that are made in his testes, the pouch of skin behind his penis. They are mixed with a white liquid called semen. A woman has eggs inside her body, in her ovaries. When parents make a baby, the semen comes from the dad's penis and takes the sperm to the mother's womb. One of the sperms will go into the egg, and that is the very beginning of a new baby who will grow in the mother's belly." The answer is basic and may be all the children want to know.

Other questions to prepare for include:
- How does the baby get out of Mommy's belly?
- What is sex?
- What is masturbating?
- What are wet dreams?
- What is puberty?
- What is menstruation?

Answers should be simple and basic.

Questions about transgenderism, homosexuality, and other similar topics may come up because of what your children see in school, or even out in public. Be prepared to give a simple explanation of this as well. The dangers and damaging effects of pornography should be mentioned too.

Situations in everyday life have many teachable moments. Nature can help start important conversations. Seeing animals feeding their babies can teach your children about mothers having milk to provide for their babies, and how it is the same for humans because of God's knowledge of our needs. Animals try to attract the opposite sex by (birds) fluffing their feathers, or letting off certain scents, and other methods of attraction. Humans also try to attract the opposite sex by practicing good hygiene, taking care of their bodies, being kind, and all sorts of other practices.

Sharing your own years of going through puberty can help your own children because they will know that you understand, and that what they are going through is normal and will turn out fine.

Let's move on to the final age group and book of this three-part series!

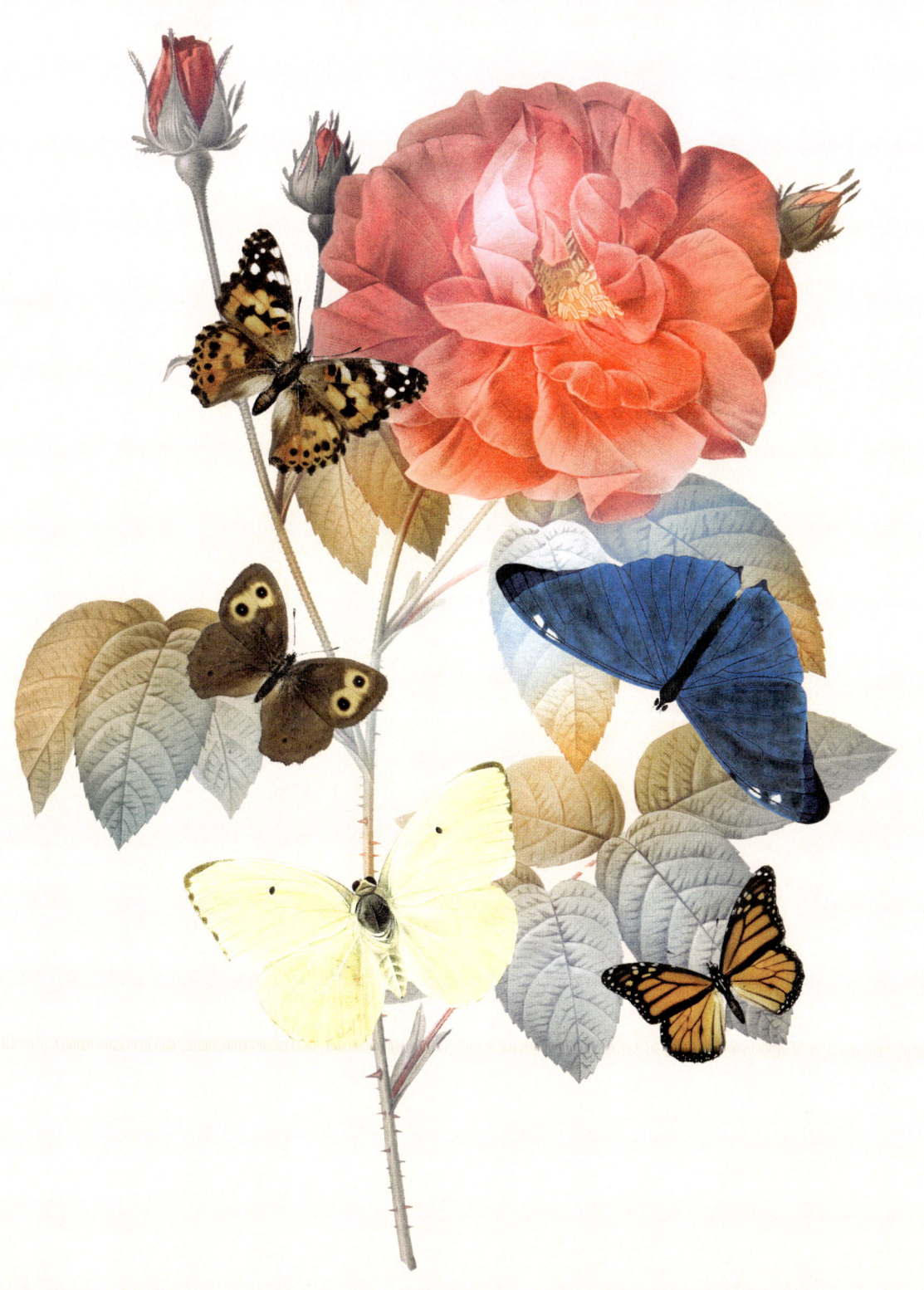

FACTS OF LIFE 9

Unit 1
WHAT TEENS SHOULD KNOW ABOUT THEIR BODIES AND SEXUAL IDENTITY

Today's culture is quite different from what it was twenty years ago. Society has introduced some very dangerous ideas to young people, gaining advocates to push and support alternate lifestyles that are damaging our youth in irreversible ways. Your diligence as a parent is crucial in helping your children mature into healthy adults who are not permanently harmed by these worldly agendas.

Transgenderism is a growing lifestyle, currently affecting approximately 300,000 young people. The definition of a transgender person is one who identifies as something other than the sex they were born with. Many young people are in different stages of transitioning, which is defined as changing from one form (in this case, sex) to another.

The transgender lifestyle has been advertised as something to celebrate and embrace as a brave move by those who are confused about their true identity, and believe they were mistakenly born as the wrong sex. Some people also identify as non-binary, which is a belief that they do not identify with either sex.

Many other terms relate to alternate lifestyles, including genderqueer, agender, gender fluid, lesbian, gay, bisexual, and more. Millions of students attend schools that are adopting policies to placate those pushing transgender ideology and related alternative lifestyles.

Your engagement with your teens on topics related to transgenderism will help them to see truths that are ignored or hidden from the public eye. Young people may not understand why these things are issues at all, but a closer look reveals many things that will reassure them that God knows what He is doing and that He does all things well.

The psalmist, David, wrote in Psalm 139:13-16: "For you created my inmost being; you knit me together in my mother's womb. I praise you because I am fearfully and wonderfully made; your works are wonderful, I know that full well. My frame was not hidden from you when I was made in the secret place, when I was woven together in the depths of the earth. Your eyes saw my unformed body; all the days ordained for me were written in your book before one of them came to be."

Rather than accepting children and teen's beliefs that they were born the wrong sex because they like hobbies and activities normally enjoyed by the opposite sex, embracing diversity is the healthy solution.

LOOKING AT THE FACTS

Some statistics related to transgender issues are:

- Transgender youth have higher levels of suicidal behaviors than their peers.[1]
- Children with gender dysphoria under the age of 18 are undergoing surgeries to alter their breasts and genitals.[2]
- Approximately 80% of children with gender confusion become comfortable with their birth gender as they get older.[3]
- Infertility affects most people who transition.[4]
- Females who have testosterone treatments are at risk of cancer[5]

While many people are referring to human beings as being on a gender spectrum, this is an idea that is not based on fact. A person's sex is not on a fluctuating scale. Facts include:

- Sex is determined at conception. It is not "assigned" at birth. It is determined by the body's reproductive organs. Chromosomes present a person's sex: XY (male) and XX (female). Chromosomes are part of nearly every cell in the human body, including hair and teeth.

- A person's sex is not determined by feelings. It is biologically proven to be one sex or the other. Those who identify as transgender do so by self-proclamation.

- Having abnormalities in the sexual organs is called DSD, which stands for Disorder of Sexual Development. Most abnormalities are specific to one sex or the other. They do not create

Unit 1
WHAT TEENS SHOULD KNOW ABOUT THEIR BODIES AND SEXUAL IDENTITY

a third sex. Having a DSD does not mean a person is transgender. Most people with this disorder do not identify as transgender. Additionally, most transgender people do not have DSDs.

- Autism and mental disorders are both common in people with gender dysphoria.
- Studies show that up to 98% of children with gender dysphoria will outgrow their desire to transition if medications and surgeries have not interfered with their natural growth.[6]
- Children as young as 13 years old have had body-altering surgeries for the purpose of transitioning.[7] Professionals are being pressured to accept a child's belief that they were born the wrong sex.[8]
- Many complications can happen from sex reassignment surgeries, including hormonal imbalances, blood clots, and infection. This also puts the recipients at higher risk of cardiovascular related death.
- Friendship circles of young people that have transgender people in them have seen rapid developments of gender dysphoria in other young people in the circle.
- Data shows that suicide has been considered by over 80% of transgender people and 40% have actually attempted to end their lives. The highest rate of suicide in transgender people is among the youth.[10] Depression and anxiety are also common struggles.
- Many people who have transitioned have also reported that it did not help their gender dysphoria and realized the dysphoria was connected to other issues in their lives, including trauma and sexual abuse.[11]

BETTER ALTERNATIVES

Instead of shaming or bullying children and teens who do not fit into stereotypes for their birth sex, accepting a child's unique interests allows the child to be expressive without pressure about their sexuality at a young age.

In scripture, Paul's statement in 1 Corinthians 13:11 says: "When I was a child, I talked like a child, I thought like a child, I reasoned like a child..." Childhood includes exploration of new things, using one's imagination, developing physically and emotionally, and many other things.

Boys who like shopping and cooking are still 100% boys, even if most of their male friends participate in woodwork and baseball. Girls who like mud and bugs are still 100% girls, even when their female friends like tea parties and sparkly shoes.

Allowing children to be children without complicating matters with ideas of transgenderism at young ages gives them opportunities to enjoy childhood much more, rather than persuading them, or allowing them to be persuaded, to believe they were born the wrong sex.

The majority of children and teens with gender dysphoria are struggling with additional issues, which include trauma and sexual abuse. Many who go through medical procedures for transitioning later realize their actions were carried out because of misunderstanding of their true needs. Praying, finding mental health care, and giving emotional support for the actual underlying issues will help those young people far more, and will also benefit them as they mature and learn to handle other issues in life.

Many people are not aware of God's desires or commands for humanity. Because of this, people are using human reasoning to try to fix issues of the heart - the heart that God created and knows how to completely satisfy.

God's desires for mankind are drastically different from what is seen in society on a daily basis. Sometimes this is by choice, but often it is because people have little knowledge about the ways of God. The Bible says in Isaiah 55:8-9: "For my thoughts are not your thoughts, neither are your ways my ways, saith the Lord. For as the heavens are higher than the earth, so are my ways higher than your ways, and my thoughts than your thoughts."

Unit 1

WHAT TEENS SHOULD KNOW ABOUT THEIR BODIES AND SEXUAL IDENTITY

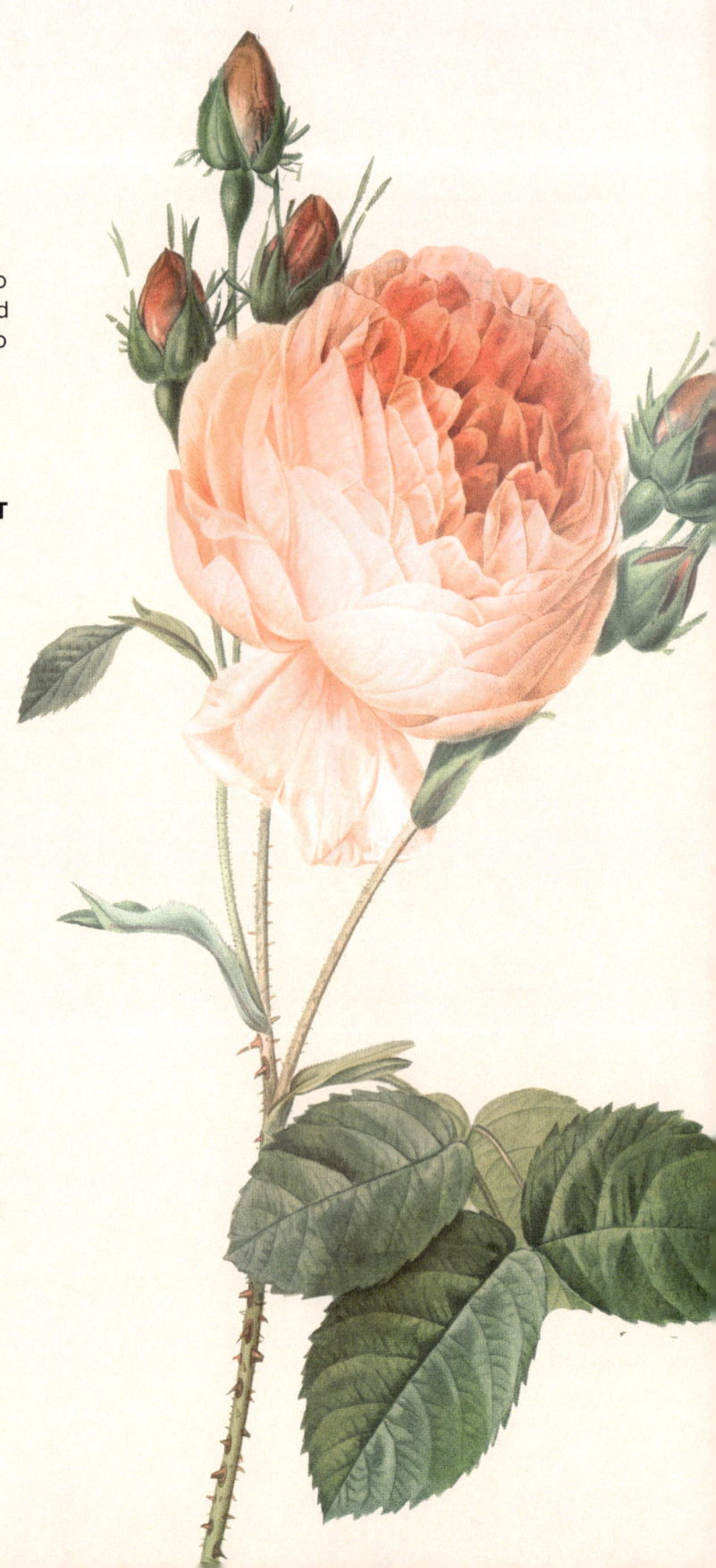

Desperate parents are grasping for solutions to help their adolescent with emotional turmoil. If your teens are struggling with ideas of being transgender, compassion coupled with counseling or mental health care can help you and your children discover the deeper issues that are present under the surface, giving you greater hope for the future. Some of those issues will include things that have happened to them, causing feelings of humiliation, anger, and other things that they feel ashamed to share. So often, young people carry the weight of other people's sins. They deserve the chance to be healed and helped from those wrongs that are impacting their own decisions.

WHY GOD'S WAYS ARE IMPORTANT WHEN IT COMES TO TRANSGENDERISM

As research and studies have revealed, young people transition for deeper reasons than wanting to be the opposite sex. Some want to disassociate from the body they were sexually abused in. Some confuse homosexual feelings with having gender dysphoria. Some feel as if they don't fit in with others and believe transitioning is the answer.

The ways of God address much more than the surface of this important topic. Before addressing the outward evidence of an inward struggle, God wants young people to know:

1. They are deeply and genuinely loved.

Romans 8:37-39 not only expounds upon God's love for us, and the inability for anything to separate us from His love, but it also lets us know that through Him, we are more than conquerors! It says: "No, in all these things we are more than conquerors through him who loved us. For I am convinced that neither death nor life, neither angels nor demons, neither the present nor the future, nor any powers, neither height nor depth, nor anything else in all creation, will be able to separate us from the love of God that is in Christ Jesus our Lord."

FACTS OF LIFE 12

Unit 1
WHAT TEENS SHOULD KNOW ABOUT THEIR BODIES AND SEXUAL IDENTITY

2. They are valuable and God has a plan for each of their lives.

"For you created my inmost being; you knit me together in my mother's womb. I praise you because I am fearfully and wonderfully made; your works are wonderful, I know that full well. My frame was not hidden from you when I was made in the secret place, when I was woven together in the depths of the earth. Your eyes saw my unformed body; all the days ordained for me were written in your book before one of them came to be." Psalm 139:13-16

3. He desires for them to come to Him and let Him help them with the heavy burdens they carry.

"Come to me, all you who are weary and burdened, and I will give you rest. Take my yoke upon you and learn from me, for I am gentle and humble in heart, and you will find rest for your souls. For my yoke is easy and my burden is light." Matthew 11:28

The God who created human beings with an amazing number of intricate details wants to free people from anxiety, depression, suicidal thoughts, and every other feeling that troubles each person's mind.

Hebrews 4:15 reminds us that, "...we do not have a high priest who is unable to empathize with our weaknesses..." Jesus walked on the earth and experienced the emotions of mankind. He relates to His creation. He knows each potential state of mind we can encounter, including the ugly, painful places our minds visit and dwell.

Jesus not only understands our emotions, but He also offers encouragement through His inspired Word. Proverbs 3:5-6 tells us to: "Trust in the Lord with all your heart and lean not on your own understanding; in all your ways submit to him, and he will make your paths straight." A heart and mind that allow Jesus to lead will find answers and guidance that will bring the desired calm that their hearts desire, and also the satisfaction that cannot be found by the humanistic ideas pushed by society.

As a parent, your affirmations that build your son's and daughter's confidence, alongside teaching them God's design for young men and young women, will help you ward off the aggressive push for the heartbreaking transgender lifestyle.

IMPORTANT NOTE

The facts included in this book can help you share some of the basic information pertaining to transgenderism. If you haven't spoken to your teens about this topic yet, we encourage you to help them to learn the facts. It can help them avoid confusion on the issue while protecting their minds and being compassionate to those who are involved in this heartbreaking lifestyle.

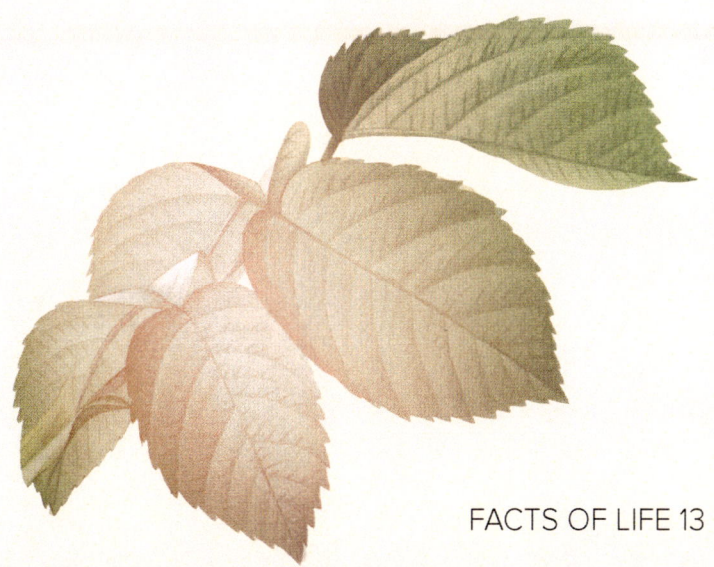

FACTS OF LIFE 13

Unit 1
WORKBOOK QUESTIONS

1. Have you seen much of the transgender movement in your teenager's schools? If so, have you talked to them about the topic?

Unit 1
WORKBOOK QUESTIONS

2. Were you aware of many of the facts shared in this book pertaining to the transgender lifestyle? Have you shared the facts with your adolescents?

Unit 1
WORKBOOK QUESTIONS

3. Have you noticed your teens questioning their self-worth, or becoming curious about the transgender lifestyle? What are some ways that you have tried to dissuade them?

Unit 1
WORKBOOK QUESTIONS

4. Whether your teens are curious about the transgender lifestyle, or are comfortable in the sex they were born with, do you find ways to continue encouraging them about their worth and the being wonderfully made by God?

Unit 2
WHAT TO EXPECT WHEN YOUR TEEN GOES THROUGH PUBERTY

This age group is when all children should be going through puberty. If your children have not started puberty by around the time they are 14 years old, speak to your doctor in case there are underlying reasons that may need medical treatment.

This age group is also more aware that puberty and sexuality are deeper subjects than what they have been taught up to this point. Throughout this book series, we have continually emphasized and encouraged you, as the parent, to assure your children that they can approach you with their questions. Conversations about puberty and sexuality should be ongoing throughout the years, just as your children's bodies continue growing and changing each year. Putting off these important conversations may cause your children to find their answers from others who may not give accurate information or who offer answers that do not share the same values you want your family to have.

WHAT TEENS SHOULD KNOW ABOUT PUBERTY

There are several things your teenager should be taught about puberty. Teens will notice changes happening in the opposite sex as well as in their own sex. You can teach them about puberty in both. Knowing that their peers will also go through puberty can help them to not feel alone.

Speak to your teens about the upcoming changes they will begin experiencing, both physically and emotionally. You should explain menstruation to your daughters before it begins. It can be frightening to see blood in their private area if they don't understand what is happening.

Several things adolescents should know about the changes in girls going through puberty are:

- The shape of their body will change. They will become rounder, especially their hips and legs.
- Their breasts will begin to grow. It is not uncommon for one side to grow larger or faster than the other. They will normally even out over time.
- They will begin menstruating. Their cycles will typically last around 3-7 days. Sanitary napkins (pads) and tampons are used to absorb the blood.
- Each month, girls have a period, and their uterine lining prepares for a fertilized egg by filling with blood. If the egg is not fertilized, the girls will have a period. If the egg is fertilized, girls will become pregnant.
- They will grow pubic and underarm hair. Additionally, the hair on their legs will grow thicker and become darker.
- They will begin to sweat more.
- They often develop acne.
- They will have a growth spurt.

Several things teens should know about the changes in boys going through puberty are:

- Their penises and testicles will grow larger.
- Their voices will change and become deeper, sometimes cracking or sounding squeaky while their larynx is growing.
- They will grow facial hair, pubic hair, and underarm hair. Additionally, the hair on their legs will grow thicker and become darker.
- Their muscles will increase in size.
- They will ejaculate in their sleep, commonly known as wet dreams.
- They will begin to sweat more.
- They often develop acne.
- They will have a growth spurt.

REASONS CHANGES HAPPEN DURING PUBERTY

Puberty is a time in your children's lives when their bodies will grow rapidly. Their brains release a certain hormone called gonadotropin-release hormone (GnRH) at a certain age, which will then reach the pituitary gland, a small gland that is located just under the brain. The gland will release two additional puberty hormones called luteinizing hormone (LH) and follicle-stimulating hormone (FSH). These hormones work differently

FACTS OF LIFE 18

Unit 2
WHAT TO EXPECT WHEN YOUR TEEN GOES THROUGH PUBERTY

in each sex. All of the changes happening inside the body of your children in this age group are changing their bodies into adults.

Growth spurts usually last about two or three years. At its peak, some young people will grow four inches or more in a single year. During puberty is the final time children will grow in height.

Body shapes will change for both boys and girls during puberty.

In girls, their hips widen to prepare their bodies to be capable of carrying and delivering babies. Weight gain in their thighs comes from the hormone estrogen. It causes an increase in fat cells that commonly form around the buttocks and thighs.

The development of breasts is caused by released hormones that cause fat to accumulate and cause growth.

Boys sometimes experience bodily growth that includes arms, legs, hands, and feet growing faster than the rest of their bodies. It can cause them to feel clumsy during this period. Their scrotum and testes will begin to grow, which happens before their penis enlarges. Their penis will begin to grow as the scrotum and testes continue to grow. These changes are the result of increased testosterone production in their bodies.

Body hair is caused by hormonal increases. Boys have higher levels of the hormone testosterone, which causes them to grow hair where girls normally do not, such as on their faces, chest, and in time, their backs.

Acne that appears during puberty is often seen on the face, upper back, and upper chest. It happens due to hormones that cause oil glands to "activate".

Body odor occurs when sweat glands become more active during puberty and give off chemicals that cause a stronger smell.

Wet dreams cause boys to ejaculate (have an orgasm) in their sleep. They begin during puberty when more testosterone is produced in their bodies and are a normal occurrence, although some boys do not have them.

Treating puberty as a special and important period of time in your children's lives can ease some of the awkwardness and anxieties they feel as their body is going through so many changes. This is a good time to emphasize the importance of self-care once again. Good food choices and cleanliness can help minimize issues like acne, body odor, and odor that can be embarrassing when girls are not practicing good hygiene during their menstrual cycles.

PUBERTY AND MOODINESS

Along with all the physical changes your children go through during puberty, there are also emotional ups and downs that will cause their moods to fluctuate quite a bit more. Their brains are also adjusting to changing hormones as their bodies are adjusting. Mood swings are another normal part of puberty. One minute, your teens may be laughing and having an enjoyable time, and, within minutes, they may become disgruntled and stomp out of the room.

When your teens go through puberty, parts of the brain become stronger, causing them to feel emotions more intensely. The area of the brain that helps regulate those emotions still needs time to develop. Because situations and seasons of life can be overwhelming, teens can feel even more out of control because they haven't yet learned how to handle emotional stress.

There are several factors that can trigger your teen's moods negatively. Some of these are:

- Hormones
- Not getting enough sleep
- Physical changes they are dealing with, causing awkwardness and self-consciousness
- Feeling scared, alone, or having anxiety

FACTS OF LIFE 19

Unit 2
WHAT TO EXPECT WHEN YOUR TEEN GOES THROUGH PUBERTY

- Pressure from school
- Pressure from peers
- Too many things going on in their lives at the same time
- Stress
- Family disagreements

Moodiness is a normal part of puberty. When it becomes frustrating to you as a parent, remember that it is also frustrating for your children. They are still learning to handle their emotions. Your patience, alongside methods to help them, can make the mood swings easier to cope with, both for you and for your children.

Things you can do to help include:

- Listening to their feelings and remaining calm. Acknowledging how they are feeling.
- Helping them understand why they might feel the way they do.
- Letting them have time alone to process how they are feeling, but being available to talk if they would like to.
- Helping your children express themselves and discover ways to help their heavier moods become lighter. Complimenting the better attitudes and behaviors.
- Helping your children learn problem-solving techniques when difficulties arise for them. This should be done with your supervision but not completely by yourself. Children need to develop problem-solving skills for life. They can succeed in making better choices with your oversight and reasoning when you help them come to good conclusions.
- Have clear rules for behavior. Allowing your child to learn through their moodiness is important, and you can help their "down" times to become less frequent. Even so, putting limitations and expectations on negative behavior is good. Allow them to be upset, but don't allow them to punch things, or say mean things, or show disrespect in the words they say to others.
- Set healthy rules for eating and sleeping in the home. Set a time for phones and video games to be turned off. Keep fresh fruits and vegetables in the home and cook more homemade meals instead of eating processed foods.

If you notice severe mood swings or prolonged times of being upset, your children may be dealing with something beyond puberty. If you notice a significant difference in your children's behavior (including their thoughts and feelings), see them behaving differently at home, school, and with friends, or notice them feeling "down" for two weeks or more, talk to your physician.

ATTRACTION, DATING, AND SEXUAL DESIRE

The pre-teen and teenage years begin introducing new feelings in your children relating to romantic relationships. These feelings are part of the many other emotions your teenagers are feeling. You will likely see many ups and downs in your children's emotions as they begin caring for others in a more intimate way.

In children 9-11, you may begin to see more independence displayed as they become more interested in friends. Feeling romantically attracted to others can usually be seen in children between the ages of 10 and 14. From the age of 15 up to adulthood, romantic relationships can become the main focus for your teenagers. While this is normal and common, there are also teens who will be more focused on their education, sports activities, or other things that interest them.

Sometime during this age range, teenagers will begin having crushes. Identity crushes are when your teen admires someone and want to be like that person. Romantic crushes are when your children have strong feelings of liking someone, usually in secret, which pass after a short time.

Your growing and changing children should not be made to feel embarrassed for feelings that are very real to them. Being available to listen to their feelings keeps an open line of communication which is extremely important in the years leading to adulthood. There are

Unit 2
WHAT TO EXPECT WHEN YOUR TEEN GOES THROUGH PUBERTY

crucial lessons happening during these years and your children need your influence.

Younger teens will usually spend time together in groups and move on to spending more time alone with someone when they feel attracted to them. The feelings your children experience are part of growing up. Helping them to set godly, healthy boundaries with their emotions and actions will prepare them for the future when they are looking for a spouse.

Today's culture considers premarital sex, multiple marriages, same-sex marriage, open marriage, having children out of wedlock, and multiple other ideas for relationships to be normal. Even though each of these situations is prevalent in society, God's plan for marriage is still the healthiest option for everyone. As a parent, no matter what your own situation is, you can influence your children to follow God's plan and include others in healthy relationships as examples and role models.

God's desire is that one man and one woman save their bodies from any sexual activity until they unite in marriage, where sexual intercourse is a gift the couple gives to each other. It is during the commitment of marriage that children can be conceived and born into a family that honors God and His ways. Parents raise their children and teach godly morals and values, working to see their children continue godly living as they bring forth the next generation.

Much more is entailed in marriage than the union of a man and woman. Godly families show love and respect, nurturing and selflessness for each other. Abuse, neglect, and denying provision and protection are not pleasing to God. A godly marriage is a blessing to both spouses and the children who become part of their beautiful union. Because so many of these negative traits are seen regularly in society, your influence with the proper view of what is good and acceptable must be seen by and taught to your children.

It is normal for your teenager to have crushes and to be romantically attracted to the opposite sex. Encourage them to build friendships with those they feel attracted to. Having boyfriends and girlfriends at ages much too early for marriage sets them up for many break-ups, which sets a pattern that can be continued once they get married. Dating should begin when a young person is ready for marriage. That may seem like a foreign concept in our society but young people who are looking for their spouse will not view dating as a casual hobby that could lead to a great deal of hurt and temptation.

When your adolescent children are at an age and maturity level that you believe they are ready to make plans for commitment and marriage, take some time to give them guidelines that will help them and protect them. Help them recognize unhealthy personality traits in the opposite sex and remind them to respect and protect their bodies as you have been teaching them for years. Build your son's and daughter's self-worth as they enter this time in their lives.

Being sexually attracted to the person you are considering for marriage is normal. God intended sex to be something good and enjoyable within a marriage commitment. Encourage your children to reserve their bodies for marriage, even though they may experience temptation. Being pressured by their boyfriend or girlfriend is a red flag. It may seem overboard to some; however, there are young people who do not give full-body hugs or kiss their spouses-to-be until they are married. Talk to your teen about temptations and explore solutions and preventative measures they can follow, such as group dating, being home by a certain time, etc. Point out the positive side of abstinence before marriage, such as having no regrets. Purity before marriage is one of many ways to express our love and devotion to God as we follow His will and desire for marriage.

When your teens make mistakes in regard to sexuality and abstinence, they need to know your love for them has not wavered, and that they can find restoration and grace for the future. One mistake does not need to become a habit that controls their future actions.

FACTS OF LIFE 21

Unit 2
WHAT TO EXPECT WHEN YOUR TEEN GOES THROUGH PUBERTY

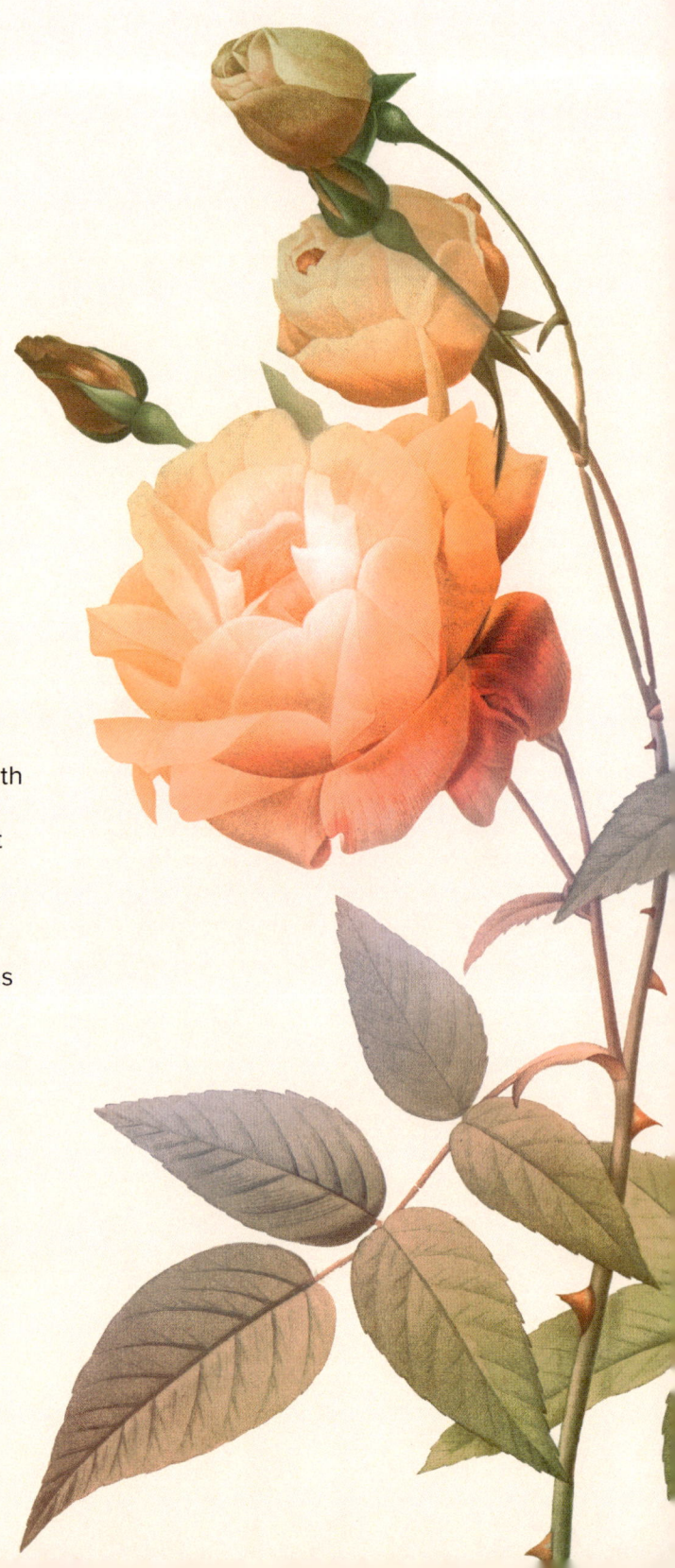

MASTURBATION

Masturbation is a highly sensitive topic that can cause shame or embarrassment if not handled correctly. This may feel like a difficult subject to discuss, but, as with other areas of sexuality, you as the parent are the best person to talk to your child about it. Let them know you are a safe place for them to bring their questions anytime.

When conversations arise that are openings to talk about the subject, you can ask your children what they know about masturbation. You can correct any misinformation they have and give them a basic explanation about it. Use proper terms without being too graphic.

Explain that masturbation is when your teens touch their own genitals until they feel sexual arousal. It is not damaging to the genitals or the body and is something very common among teenagers. The urges this age group feels are part of normal development. Orgasm is something that may occur during masturbation.

Teenagers should further understand that there can be problematic behaviors that go along with masturbation: using pornography, fantasizing, or doing it when others are with them. It can also be emotionally harmful when used as a tool to cope with difficulties and stress. They should be taught that masturbating with their boyfriend or girlfriend is not a healthy practice for abstinence before marriage and can negatively impact healthy marital intimacy.

Encourage your teens to focus on other things during times of stress, boredom, and other emotions that cause them to desire to masturbate, but also teach them not to worry excessively if they do masturbate. Encourage them to participate in other enjoyable activities, such as hobbies, sports, hanging out with friends, and other favorite pastimes. Sexual energy is not evil or bad. It is part of human nature. However, God does desire that they use their sexual energy properly, not allowing sexual urges to control their lives. Sexual intimacy with a husband or wife is a blessing within love and a committed relationship. This truth should be encouraged when discussing masturbation.

FACTS OF LIFE 22

Unit 2
WORKBOOK QUESTIONS

1. What noticeable changes have you seen in your teenagers during this time of puberty? Do you have regular conversations with your teenagers about the changes?

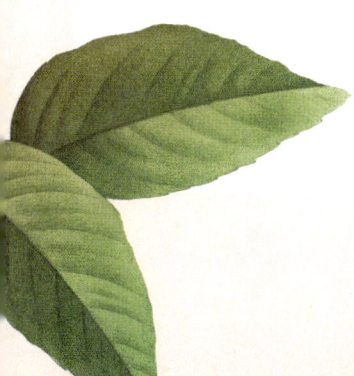

Unit 2
WORKBOOK QUESTIONS

2. Are your teenagers displaying the common moodiness in this age group? Have you talked to your teenagers about methods of coping and improving how they feel?

Unit 2
WORKBOOK QUESTIONS

3. Have your teens started showing romantic interest in the opposite sex? What conversations have you had about dating, sexual feelings, and masturbation? Do they feel comfortable talking to you about these topics? What are some ways you can encourage them to come to you about these very sensitive matters?

Unit 3
SEXUAL BEHAVIOR IN TEENS

Teenage children are at a point in life when their bodies are going through rapid changes as adulthood is approaching within the next few years of their lives. This is when you will want to talk to your teens about the deeper details of sexuality.

If you've had an ongoing conversation with your children over the years, they will already have some basic knowledge about sex. This is the age group where you will bring all of the information together to present the whole picture of intimacy and sexual activity.

DIFFERENT FORMS OF SEX

There are several different ways that people perform sexual acts. The list below gives a brief description of the different forms of sex:

- **Vaginal sex** is when a man inserts his penis in a woman's vagina and moves in and out and around the vagina entrance, causing arousal. The stimulation and sexual pleasure felt in the genitals will cause the bodies to have orgasms, which is an intense feeling that is considered the peak of sexual pleasure. This is usually followed by ejaculation of semen from the penis.
- **Oral sex** is when people use their mouths to stimulate another person's genitals through sucking, licking and kissing.
- **Anal sex** is when a sex toy or a man's penis is inserted into the anus (the butt).
- **Masturbation** is when people use their hands to sexually arouse their genitals or their partner's genitals.
- **Fingering or a "hand job"** is when people use their hands to sexually stimulate another's genitals.
- **Dry humping or genital rubbing** is when two people rub or grind their genitals together while being at least partially clothed. There is no penetration in dry humping.
- **Group sex** is sexual intercourse that involves more than two people.
- **Phone sex** is when a phone call is used for a sexually explicit conversation that causes arousal in one or both participants, often accompanied by masturbation.
- **Sexting and online sex** means using phone calls, texts, chat rooms on the internet, email, video chat, and instant messaging to send and receive sexual chat, sexually graphic pictures, and sexually graphic videos.

This list does not talk exclusively about healthy sexual practices but gives brief descriptions to be informative. Several forms of sex do not fit into God's model of what sexual intimacy was meant to be. Sex outside of God's design can also lead to sexually transmitted diseases.

God intended sex to be an intimate gift of love between a husband and wife in marriage. He wants our bodies and our hearts to remain pure when entering marriage. Things like sexting, dry humping, and using their hands or mouth to sexually stimulate their partner's genitals may technically allow your teens to say they are pure (in the sense of not having had sexual intercourse), but these practices tear down personal boundaries and respect for each other's bodies.

Teach your teens to respect and protect their boyfriend or girlfriend by conducting themselves in ways that allow them to continually see their companion with purity.

Young people may be ignorant of the fact that sexting is illegal when it involves distributing images of minors under 18 years old. This is true even if the minor consents to having their picture shared.

PREMARITAL SEX

This series has covered the blessings of sexual pleasure in marriage as a gift from God. Husbands and wives share their bodies with each other in a lifelong commitment of monogamy, which further strengthens and blesses their marriage union.

While you teach your teenagers God's design for marriage and families, teaching them the consequences of premarital sex can encourage them during times of temptation.

FACTS OF LIFE 26

Unit 3
SEXUAL BEHAVIOR IN TEENS

Society has promoted premarital sex as normal, acceptable behavior. Feelings of wanting intimacy and sex itself are not bad things, but done in a different order than what God intended creates many issues for those who participate in premarital sex.

Some of the consequences of premarital sex include:

- **Giving up a priceless gift.** While God offers forgiveness and redemption, having sex with someone before marriage is not something that can be erased physically. Virginity cannot be given back. (This does not refer to those who have been victims of sexual abuse. Victims who do not share their bodies willingly with others until marriage still have a precious gift to give to their spouse.)
- **Regret and loss of self-respect.**
- Confusion. When couples partake in premarital sex, emotions of love and physical intimacy can get confused. The chemical oxytocin is released during sex and bonds people on hormonal and emotional levels. This can prolong unhealthy relationships.
- **Unplanned pregnancy.** This becomes a life-altering challenge for unmarried young people. Many times, young ladies find themselves single once they become pregnant. Every baby born is precious. Even so, young people faced with an unplanned pregnancy must alter future plans to accommodate becoming parents. Furthermore, many unplanned pregnancies end in abortion, which has lasting emotional remorse for the young mothers who choose this option.
- **Sexually transmitted diseases.**
- **Loss of the intended specialness.** Viewing sex casually during the dating years causes its specialness to diminish. It can further cause a lack of respect for those who freely share their bodies with others.

SEXUALLY TRANSMITTED DISEASES

Sexually transmitted diseases (STDs), also called sexually transmitted infections (STIs), are infections that get passed from one person to another through sexual contact. There are more than 20 types of sexually transmitted diseases, some of which carry serious consequences if they are not treated, including blindness, infertility, birth defects, paralysis, liver failure, cancer, and even death.

Some of the most common STDs and their descriptions are:

- Chlamydia, a bacterial infection in the genital tract.
- Gonorrhea, also a bacterial infection in the genital tract.
- Trichomoniasis, an infection caused by a parasite.
- Human immunodeficiency virus, known as HIV, an infection that lessens the body's ability to fight off viruses, bacteria, and fungi, which can lead to AIDS, which is life-threatening.
- Genital herpes, a virus that enters the body through mucous membrane or small tears in the skin.
- Human papillomavirus, known as HPV, an infection that can cause genital warts. Some forms of HPV cause women to be at high risk of cervical cancer.
- Hepatitis A, B, and C, all contagious viral infections that can cause the liver to become inflamed.
- Syphilis, a bacterial infection that affects your genitals, skin, and mucous membranes. It can also affect several other parts of the body, including the heart and brain.

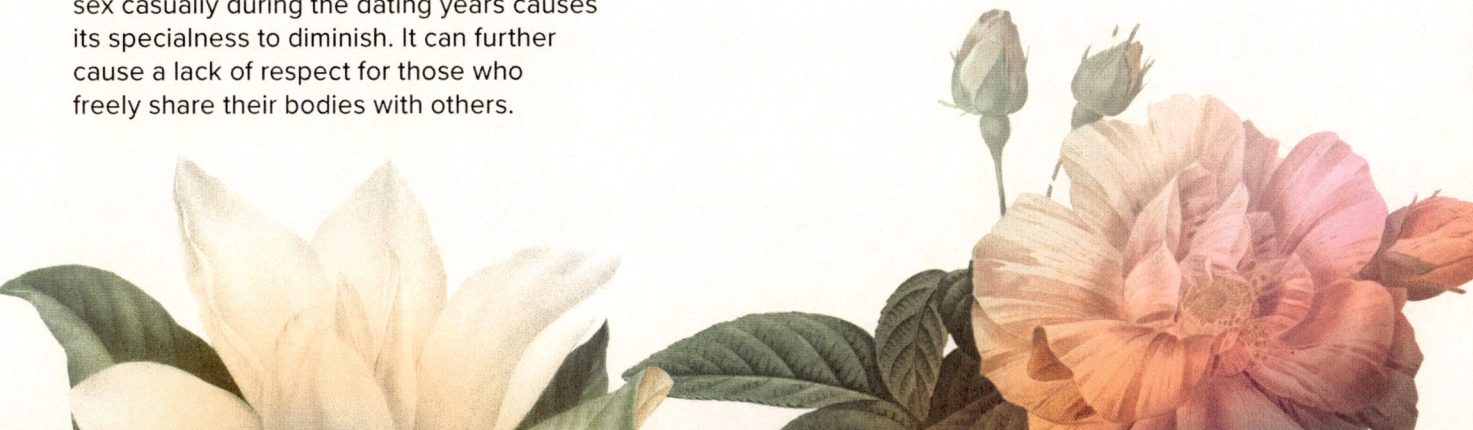

Unit 3
SEXUAL BEHAVIOR IN TEENS

SAME-SEX ATTRACTION

Even when you raise your children with godly values and teach them God's design for families, there is still the possibility that you will face the challenge of your children feeling same-sex attraction. The first unit in this book talks about these feelings sometimes coming from the popular trend in society. If that is not the case with your children, here are some guidelines to help you and your children.

As with any and every other conversation you have with your children, remaining calm and approachable will help you and your children have open communication about this subject. Many gender and sexuality-type lifestyles that differ from God's plan are demonstrated, experimented with, and are being praised culturally. This includes same-sex attraction which is seen publicly and in schools. Children should not be scolded or shut down when asking questions or experiencing emotions that are prevalent all around them. Honest answers and guidance from you are necessary, coupled with your children's knowledge of your unconditional love for them, no matter what they are facing.

Same-sex attraction does not always focus on sexuality. The attraction for boys often has to do with admiration for masculinity. They may feel envious of others that model what they want to be. Affirm your sons' masculinity and have discussions about what manhood truly is.

Girls may feel same-sex attraction because of their desire to connect with others and to have inner femininity. Speak affirming words to your daughters and encourage discussions about true femininity.

If your teen opens up to you about having same-sex attractions, allow them to express their feelings with you. They may have feelings of confusion or shame, or a confident stance for how they feel and what they want. Discourage your teen from experimenting sexually as a way to discover if they are gay or lesbian.

Ask questions.
- When did you start feeling attracted to other boys/girls?
- How often do you feel this way?
- Have you felt any attraction to the opposite sex?
- Why do you think you are gay/a lesbian?

These conversations may last for several weeks or months. Don't demand that your teen change their feelings overnight. Doing so could result in unresolved issues, and healthy, open conversations to cease.

You may want to consider asking your teenagers to speak to a Christian counselor who shares your beliefs about God's desire for marriage and families.

PORNOGRAPHY

Because access to pornography has become much easier with technology, most children will be exposed, whether purposefully or accidentally, during their teen years. This vice of entertainment or sexual indulgence is harmful in several ways.

Many young people find themselves addicted to pornography. Addiction does not only store the images in the brain but causes other difficulties. Users of pornography develop poor attitudes and unrealistic expectations for their partners. Pornography also normalizes aggression and verbal abuse while portraying women who enjoy being mistreated. Those who learn about sexuality from pornography get false impressions of what normal relationships are like.

It is not uncommon to hear of those with pornography addiction struggling with their relationships. Unfaithfulness and intimacy are also common problems among pornography users. Teenage promiscuity and pregnancy rates are also higher among pornography users in youth. Negative emotions increase when pornography users fall deeper and deeper into participation. Additionally, loneliness, problems with depression, anxiety, self-consciousness of their own bodies, and lack of self-worth also find their way into the addict's mind.

Talk to your teenagers about pornography. Explain the negative consequences of pornography and actions that relate to it, and use scientific knowledge, statistics, and reported facts on the topics you are discussing. You may want to talk about how sexual images stimulate

Unit 3
SEXUAL BEHAVIOR IN TEENS

hormones that can lead to addiction, how many pornographic websites are on the internet, how much people watch per day, and the impact it is having on changing people's personalities.

Ask your teens questions and have discussions about the topic. Some ideas for conversation are:

Tell your adolescent that many young people look at pornography to learn about sex, but many things they see are not accurate. Tell them you will give them honest answers for any questions they may have.

Get their input on ways to protect your home and family from seeing pornography.

Ask them what they think they should do if a friend shows them pornography, or if pornography pops up on a website while they are doing homework research or watching videos.

Tell them that some young people watch pornography when they are bored, lonely, just want to veg, or are feeling stressed, and then have a hard time stopping themselves from future viewings. Ask them what some good activity choices are when they feel any of those emotions.

Ask your teens what they think growing up, falling in love, and getting married will be like. Ask if they think things would be different if they or their spouse became addicted to pornography and why.

Your guidance will help guide your daughters and sons toward having healthy thinking about the topic.

You may discover your teens have already viewed pornography, or even have an addiction. If this happens, begin taking action immediately. Counseling and therapy coupled with strong support from you as the parent will help them to recover. We also offer a healing study for teens addicted to pornography called **Hearten**. Visit us at treesofhope.org to learn more. Having them step away from computers and cell phones is strongly advised.

There are also highly rated internet filters should also be installed on computers and cell phones in the home. Some choices you can look into are:

- Covenant Eyes
- Bark
- Aura
- Truple
- X3Watch
- Ever Accountable

IMPORTANT NOTE

Does your home have any sexual issues that can cause confusion or disregarded teaching for your children, such as an extramarital affair or pornography addiction? The heart of every loving parent desires to see their children succeed in life and do well emotionally and physically. Loving parents should also consider their own situations and seek help when they are dealing with struggles they are hoping to help their children avoid. If you are battling addiction or other harmful sexual issues, please reach out to someone who can help you because you are a worthy human being too.

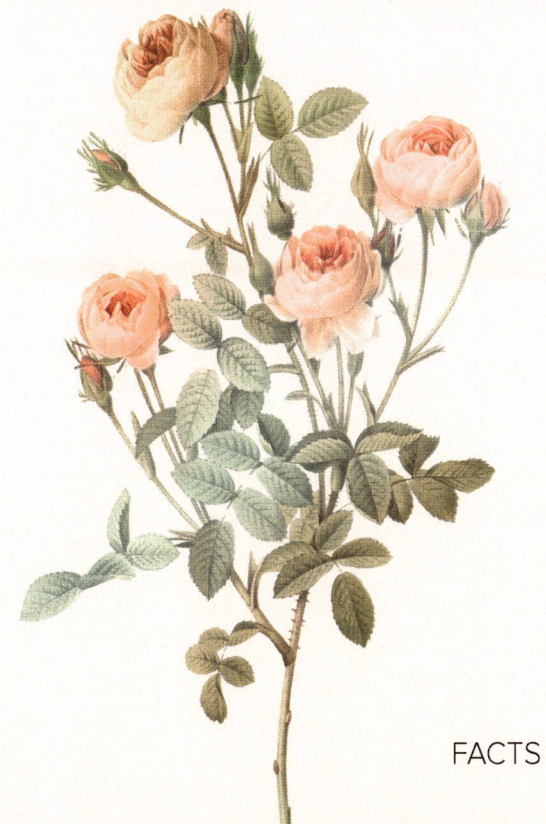

FACTS OF LIFE 29

Unit 3
WORKBOOK QUESTIONS

1. On topics of sexuality, do you feel that your answers have been knowledgeable enough to adequately inform your teens and answer any additional questions they may ask? If the answer is no, take some time to broaden your own understanding and let your teens know that you will research any questions that you do not know the answers to, and will get back to the questions soon.

Unit 3
WORKBOOK QUESTIONS

2. Talking to your teenagers about premarital sex, do you feel their previous views showed an understanding of your family values and God's design for marriage? Has abstinence been presented as a desirable boundary to them?

Unit 4
TEACHING YOUR TEENS HOW TO RESPECT THEIR BODIES & OTHERS'

People with healthy human relationships have respect for themselves and for others. They show honor and consideration to those around them, valuing others and themselves. Teaching your teens to respect others and practicing healthy boundaries will benefit them in several areas of life. This unit will cover two areas that take up large portions of youths' lives.

RESPECT IN DATING RELATIONSHIPS

The ages of dating are a special time in young people's lives when their desire for finding love and commitment awakens. Because you are teaching your teenagers God's design for marriage and family, helping them to set up boundaries for dating will help them practice healthy boundaries.

You can begin talks about serious dating relationships before your teens are in a relationship with someone. Ask them questions and share some of your own experiences. Ask questions like:

- What does dating mean to you?
- What do you think a dating relationship should look like?
- What are important factors in the person you date? Are looks important? Cleanliness? Wealth? Christian values? The same interests?
- What red flags are serious enough for someone to end a relationship?
- How does God feel about Christians dating those who are not Christians? Why is this important?
- What personality traits are important to look for in a companion?
- How much time should dating couples spend together? Should they have friends outside of each other? Should they have separate interests and hobbies?
- Is jealousy a good or bad thing?
- Should dating couples tell each other what they can and cannot do, such as get together with friends, go on a family vacation, or buy themselves a new outfit?
- What physical boundaries do you think are important? Do you think kissing is acceptable? Making out? Touching each other in sexual ways as long as you don't have sex?
- Why is it hard to talk about sex?
- What are the right reasons to have sex? What are the wrong reasons?

You can add additional questions that you feel are important to help guide your teens.

Before your teens begin a relationship, encourage them to write out their emotional and physical boundaries. It is easier to think things through and set healthy limits for their beliefs and actions before their emotions are involved. Young people should think about affection and physical contact beforehand. What are good boundaries in this area that will help them remain pure before marriage? What will help them avoid temptation? When is kissing OK?

GUIDELINES FOR DATING

There are several actions your teens can take to help them stay on the right path when they are dating. Talk to them about the following ideas, encourage them to implement them, and involve the young man or young woman they are dating.

Encourage your teens to:

- **Discuss physical boundaries early in the relationship.** This may seem awkward but making boundaries clear from the beginning can save your teens frustration and heartache. If your teens want to save sexual intimacy for marriage and the person they are dating thinks of sex as something casual to partake in if two people like each other, this is a serious issue that can help them realize they may not be a good fit.
- **Refrain from saying "I love you" too quickly.** Tell them not to become emotionally dependent on the person they are dating.

FACTS OF LIFE 32

Unit 4
TEACHING YOUR TEENS HOW TO RESPECT THEIR BODIES & OTHERS'

A companion should not be the whole source of another person's happiness. It is important to be fulfilled in their own lives. Dating should feel enjoyable but not emotionally necessary.

- **Be accountable.** Encourage your teens to remind their partners of their commitment to God whenever they feel tempted to cross over their boundaries. They can also ask you or a friend to help them with accountability by weekly conversations about their relationships and struggles.

- **Stay away from situations that can become tempting.** This can include dating during the day instead of at night, keeping a curfew, group dating, and spending time in public more than in isolation.

- **Dress modestly.** Young men and young women are both capable of dressing seductively, causing their partners to become tempted in sexual ways. Dressing modestly is a way they can show their partners that they don't want to cause them to struggle with impure thoughts.

- **Have Christian mentors or role models to talk to and view as examples.** Young married couples can be great influences on young dating couples.

- **Take things seriously if boundaries are ignored.** A partner who ignores boundaries is lacking respect for the one they claim to care about or love. This is not acceptable behavior and can even be considered sexual assault depending on the situation. Encourage your teens to come to you immediately if this happens to them.

RESPECT ON SOCIAL MEDIA AND THE INTERNET

More than ever, young people are online. Between social media platforms and online school, a great deal of their time is used interacting with others. Lead by example and help your teens understand and practice respectful and good online behavior.

Teach your teens good online behavior in the following areas:

Bullying. This is a big issue that results in depression, anxiety, low self-esteem, and even suicide for the victims. Talk to your teens about respecting how others feel and consider the feelings of others who face online bullying.

If you learn that your teens have been involved in bullying others, talk to them about their unacceptable behavior. Insist they remove any and all malicious comments and information shared online, along with a public, online apology. The bullied person should also receive an apology, either in person or in writing.

If your child is on the receiving end of bullying, help them take measures to ignore and block those who are harassing them. Print off any threatening or harassing messages your child receives and get law enforcement involved when necessary. Continue building your teenagers self-confidence.

Kindness and respect. Internet communication has caused many people to become bold and insulting because they can hide behind a screen. Sadly, this is an everyday occurrence among adults who should be setting a good example for young people by the way they interact with others online. Teach your teens that this is not acceptable, even from adults.

Young people should be taught that there are many different opinions expressed online, many of which they will not agree with. They should know it's okay to have different opinions, and it is even okay to talk about those differences if done respectfully. Name-calling, insults, threats, or any other negative behavior are never acceptable.

Sharing others' information and photos. Sharing others' exciting news or beautiful photos may seem like a perfectly good thing to do. Even so, teach your teens to ask permission first. Some people may only tell select friends information they would like to keep private.

FACTS OF LIFE 33

TEACHING YOUR TEENS HOW TO RESPECT THEIR BODIES & OTHERS'

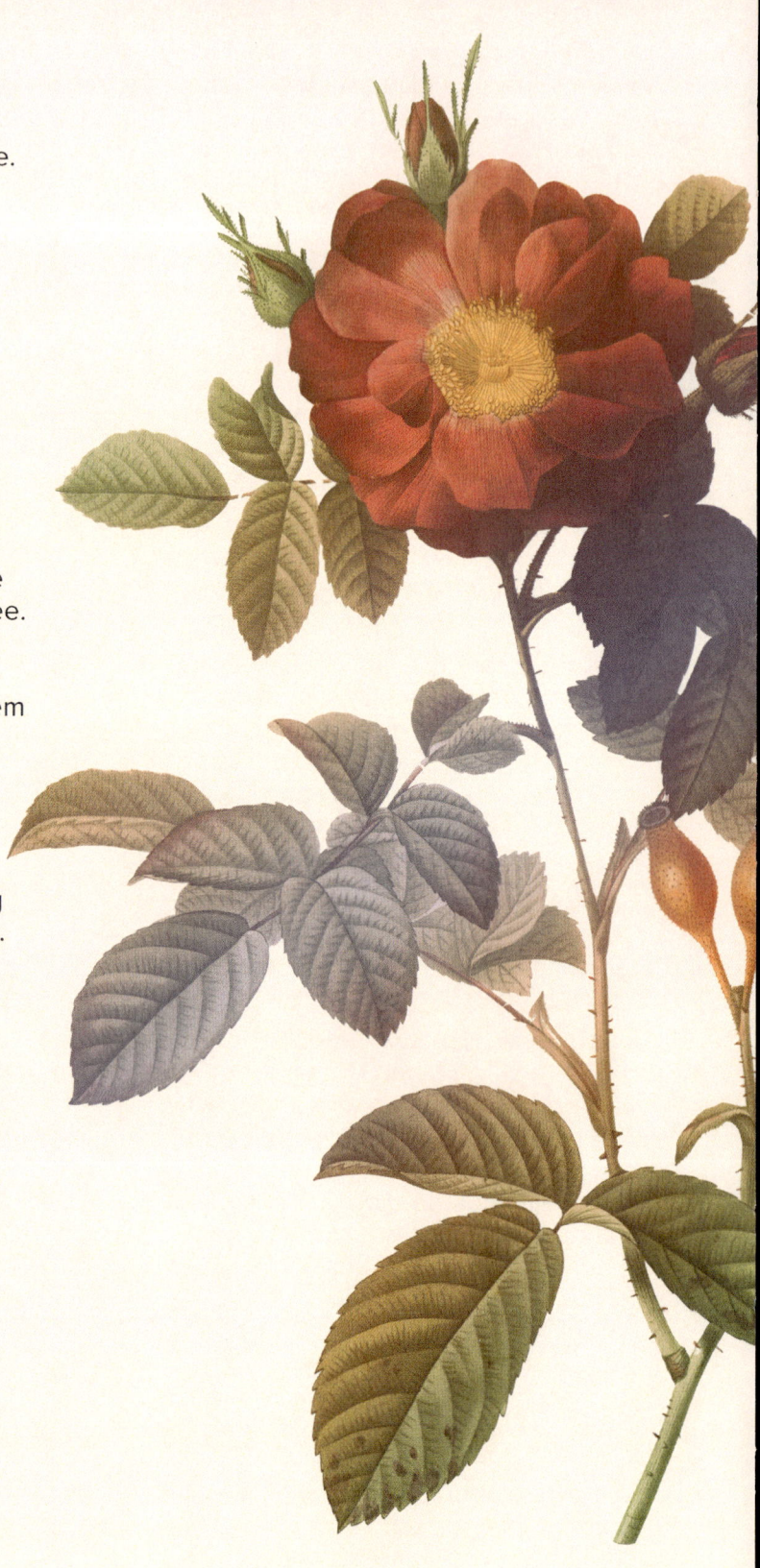

Others may not be happy to have others sharing their personal photos, especially those who try to keep their lives semi-private.

Under no circumstances should teens share photos that can embarrass, humiliate, or shame others. This includes photos that are personal and private.

Teach your teens to think about what they want to share before hitting the "post" button. Taking screenshots is common among internet users, and therefore posts can be captured before they have second thoughts and delete something they posted.

Side note: We covered information about the damaging effects of pornography in unit three. Encourage your teens to protect their minds and show themselves self-respect by never partaking in pornography usage. Remind them that they are special and that God wants to protect their hearts and minds from things that will impact their futures. Remind them that God's design for marriage is beautiful, and pornography can give them false ideas about love and relationships that are nothing like God's intentions for human relationships.

Additionally, the world of pornography has many actors and actresses who feel stuck in their situation of performing sex acts in front of the camera. The sex industry is anything but glamorous. It is a prison for the performers who don't know how to escape. Teach your youngsters to respect those who are hurt by this industry - the actors, the parents whose child performs, the brothers and sisters who can't help, and the friends who see the struggle - by not partaking in its humiliating, degrading content.

Our magazine, **Rise**, gives additional information about pornography and is available through our website.

FACTS OF LIFE 34

Unit 4
WORKBOOK QUESTIONS

1. Do you feel your teens have healthy attitudes about dating? If there are ideas you think need to be adjusted in their thinking, what ways can you help them to see things more in line with your family values?

WORKBOOK QUESTIONS

2. If you are a single parent, do you follow the guidelines you want your teens to follow? If you don't, your actions will speak louder than your words. God's design is respect and abstinence for everyone who is not married, no matter their age. He wants healthy relationships for adults as much as He does for young people.

Unit 4
WORKBOOK QUESTIONS

3. Do you model good behavior online? Self-examine yourself: Do you argue, belittle, or make fun of others and their opinions? If you do any of the above, apologize to your teens for not setting a better example. Show them your sincerity by deleting hurtful comments, apologizing where necessary, and changing your online interactions from this moment forward.

Unit 5
SEX-ED CONVERSATIONS WITH TEENS

There are many conversations to have when it comes to all things sexual. Because sexuality is on display nearly everywhere we go in society, teaching your teens about the good and bad will help them be informed. Many of those topics have been discussed in this series, and this unit will give you ideas to start conversations with your teens.

CONVERSATION STARTERS

You can take for granted that your teens already know certain things about sex, but that isn't always true. Remind your teens that you will answer all of their questions honestly when they want to learn about topics dealing with sexuality.

Here are some ideas for starting conversations about sex with your teens:

- **Talk about your own teen years.** You may not want to reveal all of your past mistakes but sharing some will show your teens that you experienced many of the same feelings they are dealing with. If you did not struggle in areas of sexual temptation during your dating years, you can share what helped you to remain sexually pure in your body and in your thoughts. If you did struggle with sexual temptations and mistakes, you can express your regret about your times of failure and tell your teens how you would do things differently and why.
- Look for teachable moments in daily life. Television shows, movies, and current events in the news offer teachable moments for many topics on sexuality, such as premarital sex, same-sex marriage, homosexuality, trangenderism, molestation, and pedophilia. Ask questions like: "Have you heard of transgenderism before? What do you think that is? What do you know about it?"
- Seeing same-sex couples holding hands in public can open a door for conversation at a later time. You can ask: "Did you notice the two women holding hands at the restaurant today? What are your thoughts? Do you know God's thoughts on same-sex couples?"
- If your teens read magazines for teenagers, take some time to look through them. Many articles talk about premarital sex without God's design for marriage included. Ask your teens if they've read the articles and ask their thoughts. Ask if the article agrees with your family's values, which are modeled after God's design for marriage.
- You can start conversations by sharing an observation. "I noticed you and Jake have been talking quite a bit." "I see you and Cindy have been spending a lot of time together after church." "I read an article recently that made me think about how much dating has changed since I was a teenager."

Try to ask mostly open-ended questions that require more than a yes or no answer. Open-ended questions help conversations to expand, which is a good thing when talking about sexuality with your teens. The more they learn from you, the less they will pick up misinformation from somewhere else.

ACTIVITIES

Activities and object lessons can be great ways to help life lessons stick in people's minds. Below are some visual and physical lessons and activities to help teens remember important lessons about sexuality.

- If you have your own special diamond, you can refer to it for this lesson. Or, you can describe the purchase of a diamond in the form of storytelling. Ask your teens why real diamonds are locked in glass cases at jewelry stores. The answer is because they are precious gems that are highly valuable. When the right buyer comes into the store and falls in love with the gem, he or she will make it their own. Because of its value, the price will be high, but completely worth it. The jeweler will remove the diamond from the glass case and put it in a small box that will be beautifully presented to the one who will cherish it forever.

FACTS OF LIFE 38

Unit 5
SEX-ED CONVERSATIONS WITH TEENS

- You can say something like: "This is just like you. You are a precious gem that God wants to protect until the time is right for you to unite with the perfect person for you. God wants you to enter into your marriage in the most special way possible. That's why He warns us to protect our minds against things like pornography, and to protect our bodies against things that will harm us both physically and emotionally. When you keep your mind and body pure until marriage, you are giving your husband/wife a gift that is so much more valuable than a diamond can ever be."

- Ask your teens to think about their favorite animal (or possibly visit a pet store). Let's use a kitten for example. Say: "Envision someone setting a kitten in front of you at 10 feet away. You aren't allowed to touch it. This far away isn't much of a problem because it is out of reach, right? What if they move the kitten to two feet in front of you? The temptation is harder, but you can still resist. What if they put the kitten on your lap and it looks up at you and begins meowing and purring, begging for your attention? Chances are, you can no longer resist. Your resistance has disappeared and you just have to pet it!"

- Then tell your teens: "This is how temptation works. When we stay far away from it, it doesn't bother us too much. When it comes to dating, being with other couples or going on dates during the day helps minimize sexual temptation. However, breaking your curfew, isolating yourselves often, and crossing your personal dating boundaries brings the temptation closer. If you break your boundaries and let your hormones get too aroused, you will find yourself in a place of physical temptation that is nearly impossible to back out of."

- Take two identical vases and break one of them into many pieces. You can do this by wrapping it in a towel and hitting it with a hammer or smashing it against a hard wooden or concrete floor. Set the intact vase next to the broken vase. Ask your teens if they can make the intact vase be like the broken vase (don't actually have them break it to show you). Next, ask them if they can make the broken vase look like the vase that is whole. The answer is no. They can glue it, but there will still be cracks and small pieces that are missing, along with other pieces that have become crumbled particles.

- Tell your teens: "Both vases represent people. Right now, you are the vase that is whole. You've protected your minds and bodies to help you remain beautiful and whole. The broken vase represents many other people who haven't protected their minds and bodies. They've allowed their minds to be filled with unclean thoughts, and they've allowed their bodies to be used by others. The truth is, the hearts of many people represented by the broken vase feel shattered (inside) too. They have regrets, insecurities, jealousies, and emotional struggles because they either didn't realize how serious the consequences of their actions would be, or they were never taught to value themselves. That's something I want to protect you from. That is why guarding your heart, mind and body are so important."

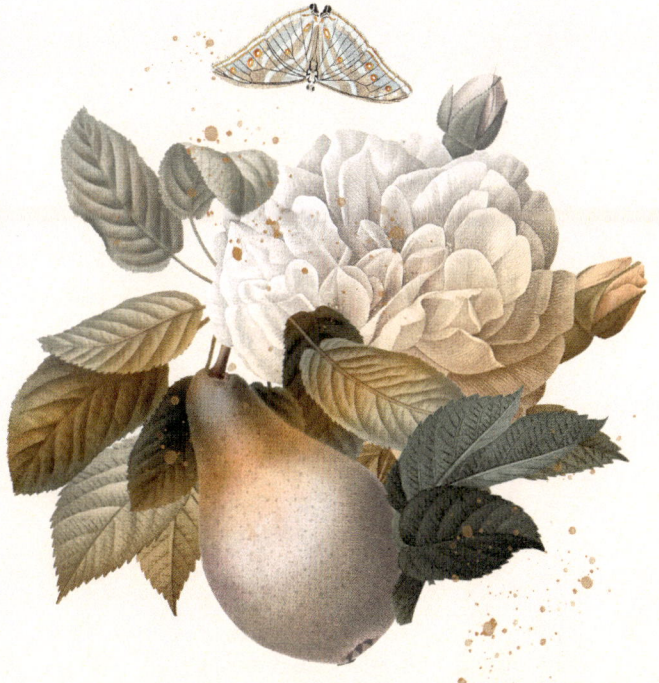

Unit 5
WORKBOOK QUESTIONS

1. What difficult topics do you think you should talk to your teens about soon? Do you feel prepared? There are many online resources to help you learn more about the complex issues of today's youth and sexuality.

Unit 5
WORKBOOK QUESTIONS

2. Were you taught any object lessons about sexuality in your teen years? Did any lessons strongly impact your views? Consider sharing them with your teenagers.

Unit 5
WORKBOOK QUESTIONS

1. After sharing the object lessons from this unit:
- Ask your teenagers if they can think of others who can help them remember how to avoid temptations.
- Use this space below and the next page to reflect on anything you learned in this unit that you want to apply immediately.
- Write out a prayer asking for God's wisdom and direction.

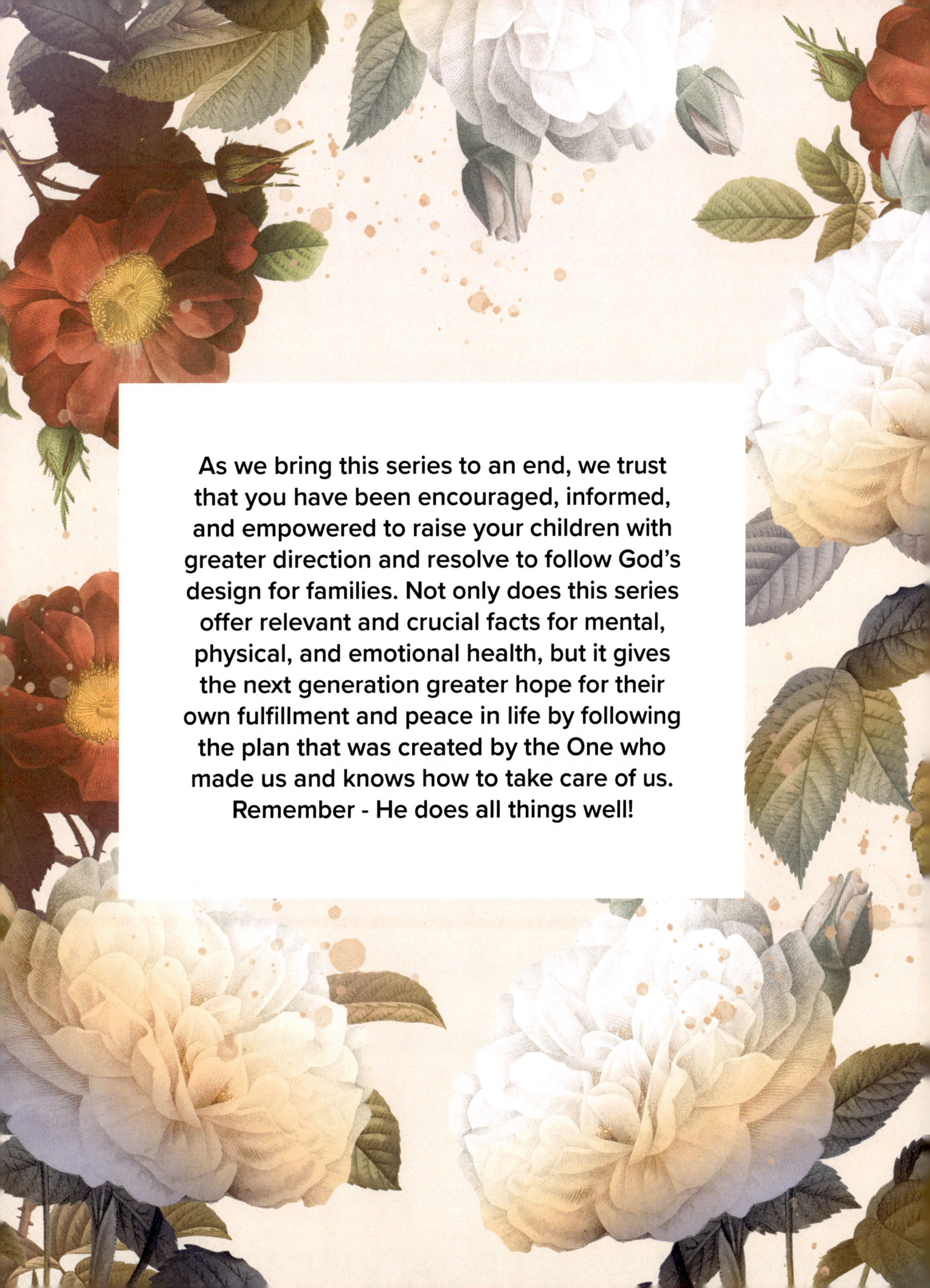

As we bring this series to an end, we trust that you have been encouraged, informed, and empowered to raise your children with greater direction and resolve to follow God's design for families. Not only does this series offer relevant and crucial facts for mental, physical, and emotional health, but it gives the next generation greater hope for their own fulfillment and peace in life by following the plan that was created by the One who made us and knows how to take care of us. Remember - He does all things well!

Citations

1. https://publications.aap.org/pediatrics/article/142/4/e20174218/76767/Transgender-Adolescent-Suicide-Behavior
2. https://www.nationalreview.com/corner/hhs-castrations-mastectomies-okay-for-transgender-minors/
3. https://fwipetitions.org/fwi/16-facts-on-gender-confusion/
4. https://endocrinenews.endocrine.org/blocking-puberty-in-transgender-youth/
5. https://endocrinenews.endocrine.org/blocking-puberty-in-transgender-youth/
6. https://academic.oup.com/jcem/article/104/3/686/5198654?login=true
7. 7. https://thefederalist.com/2018/09/12/u-s-doctors-performing-double-mastectomies-healthy-13-year-old-girls/
8. 8. https://www.theguardian.com/society/2019/jul/27/trans-lobby-pressure-pushing-young-people-to-transition
9. 9. https://journals.plos.org/plosone/article?id=10.1371/journal.pone.0202330#pone.0202330.ref045
10. 10. https://pubmed.ncbi.nlm.nih.gov/32345113/
11. 11. https://www.tandfonline.com/doi/full/10.1080/00918369.2021.1919479

Made in the USA
Middletown, DE
21 May 2024